Air Fryer Cookbook

Delicious And **Easy-To-Prepare**

Recipes **In** High Definition Pictures,

Alphabetic Table Of Contents,

And **Glossary**

Vol. 1

[5th Edition]

By

Barbara Trisler

www.MillenniumPublishingLimited.com

Table of Contents

What Is This Book All About?

This book contains proven steps and strategies on how to start preparing healthy and delicious meals that you can serve any time of the day using only one appliance – **the Air Fryer**. This innovation makes it possible to enjoy fried foods with less oil. You can also use it to whip up a wide range of dishes, snacks, and desserts.

It features loads of recipes that you can tweak in many ways to suit your preference and the availability of ingredients. Each recipe has a nutrient content guide per serving. In addition, it explains the basics about the appliance and the benefits of using it as compared to the traditional manner of frying food.

Finally, it also contains a quick guide of measurement conversion that can become handy when preparing your ingredients. Without further ado, lets get started!

Recipe Nutritional Fact Scorecard

If you'd love to receive a card that compares side-by-side the nutritional facts for all the recipes compiled in this cookbook, go to www.MillenniumPublishingLimited.com > Barbara Trisler > Recipe Nutritional Fact Scorecard

What is An Air Fryer?

An air fryer utilizes the convection mechanism in cooking food. It circulates hot air through the use of a mechanical fan to cook the ingredients inside the fryer. **The process eliminates the use of too much oil** in the traditional way of frying but still cooks food via the Maillard effect (i.e. a chemical reaction between an amino acid and a reducing sugar, usually requiring the addition of heat).

The process was named after the person who first explained it in 1912, French chemist Louis-Camille Maillard. The effect gives a distinctive flavor to browned foods, such as bread, biscuits, cookies, pan-fried meat, seared steaks, and many more.

The air fryer requires only a thin layer of oil for the ingredients to cook. It circulates hot air up to 392 degrees Fahrenheit. It's an innovative way of eliminating up to 80 percent of the oil that is traditionally used to fry different foods and prepare pastries.

You can find a dose of friendly features in air fryers depending on the brand you're using. Most brands include a timer adjustment and temperature control setting to make cooking easier and precise. An air fryer comes with a cooking basket where you'll place the food. The basket is placed on top of a drip tray. Depending on the model you're using, you will either be prompted to shake the basket to distribute oil evenly or it automatically does the job via a food agitator.

This is perfect for home use but if you're cooking for many people and you want to apply the same cooking technique, you can put your food items in specialized air crisper trays and cook them using a convection oven. An air fryer and convection oven apply the same technique in cooking but an air fryer has a smaller built and produces less heat.

How to Use Your Air Fryer

This appliance comes with a manual for easy assembly and as a handy guide for first-time users. Most brands also include a pamphlet of recipes to give you ideas about the wide range of dishes that you can create using this single kitchen appliance. Once you are ready to cook and you have all your ingredients ready, put them in the basket and insert it into the fryer. Other recipes will require you to preheat the air fryer before using. Once the basket is in, set the temperature and timer and begin cooking.

You can use an air fryer to cook food in a variety of ways. Once you get used with the basics, you can try its other features, such as advanced baking and using air fryer dehydrators.

Here are some of the cooking techniques that you can do with this single appliance:

- **Fry:** You can actually omit oil in cooking but a little amount adds crunch and flavor to your food. You can add oil to the ingredients while mixing or lightly spray the food with oil before cooking. You can use most kinds of oils but many users prefer peanut, olive, sunflower, and canola oils.

- **Roast:** You can produce the same quality of roasted foods like the ones cooked in a conventional roaster in a faster manner. This is recommended to people who need to come up with a special dish but do not have much time to prepare.
- **Bake:** There are baking pans suited for this appliance that you can use to bake bread, cookies, and other pastries. It only takes around 15 to 30 minutes to get your baked goodies done.
- **Grill:** It effectively grills your food easily and without mess. You only need to shake the basket halfway through the cooking process or flip the ingredients once or twice depending on the instructions. To make it easier, you can put the ingredients in a grill pan or grill layer with a handle, which other models include in the package or you can also buy one as an added accessory.

There are many kinds of foods that you can cook using an air fryer, but there are also certain types that are not suited for it. Avoid cooking ingredients, which can be steamed, like beans and carrots. You also cannot fry foods covered in heavy batter in this appliance.

Aside from the above mentioned, you can cook most kinds of ingredients using an air fryer. You can use it to cook foods covered in light flour or bread crumbs. You can cook a variety of vegetables in the appliance, such as cauliflower, asparagus, zucchini, kale, peppers, and corn on the cob. You can also use it to cook frozen foods and home prepared meals by following a different set of instructions for these purposes.

An air fryer also comes with another useful feature - the separator. It allows you to cook multiple dishes at a time. Use the separator to divide ingredients in the pan or basket. You have to make sure that all ingredients have the same temperature setting so that everything will cook evenly at the same time.

The Benefits of Air fryer

It is important to note that air fried foods are still fried. Unless you've decided to eliminate the use of oils in cooking, you must still be cautious about the food you eat. Despite that, it clearly presents a better and healthier option than deep frying. It helps you avoid unnecessary fats and oils, which makes it an ideal companion when you intend to lose weight. It offers a lot more benefits, which include the following:

- It is convenient and easy to use, plus, it's easy to clean.
- It doesn't give off unwanted smells when cooking.
- You can use it to prepare a variety of meals.
- It can withstand heavy cooking.
- It is durable and made of metal and high-grade plastic.
- Cooking using this appliance is not as messy as frying in a traditional way. You don't have to worry about greasy spills and stains in the kitchen.

Measurement Conversion Table

Measurement	Conversion
1 stick of butter	1/2 cup or 8 tablespoons
4 quarts	1 gallon
2 quarts	1/2 gallon
1 cup	8 fluid ounces or 1/2 pint or 16 tablespoons
2 cups	1 pint
1 quart	32 ounces or 2 pints or 4 cups
4 tablespoons	1/4 cup
8 tablespoons	1/2 cup
1/2 tablespoon	1 1/2 teaspoons
3 teaspoons	1 tablespoon

Breakfast Recipes

Air Fried Eggs

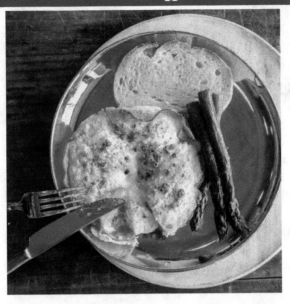

Nutritional Facts/Calories: 256 calories, 20.6g fat, 1.4g carbohydrates, 16.5g protein, 199mg cholesterol, 600mg sodium

Preparation + Cook Time: 30 minutes

Servings: 4

Ingredients:

- 1 tablespoon extra-virgin olive oil
- Salt and pepper to taste
- 4 bacon slices
- 4 eggs
- 2 cups baby spinach (rinsed and drained)
- 1/2 cup shredded cheddar cheese (divided)

Instructions:

1. Heat oil in a pan over medium-high flame. Put the spinach and cook until wilted. Transfer to a plate and drain excess liquid. Transfer them into 4 greased ramekins.

2. Add a slice of bacon and egg to each ramekin. Sprinkle cheese on top. Season with salt and pepper.

3. Arrange the ramekins inside the cooking basket of the Air Fryer. Cook for 15 minutes at 350 degrees.

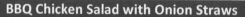

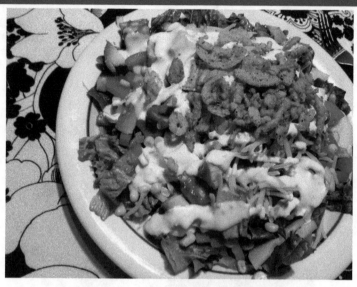

Nutritional Facts/Calories: 683 calories, 19.7g fat, 74.3g carbohydrates, 57.4g protein, 126mg cholesterol, 974mg sodium

Preparation + Cook Time: 35 minutes

Servings: 4

Ingredients:

- 3 green onions (chopped)
- 12 grape tomatoes (sliced)
- 1 cup Monterey Jack cheese (shredded)
- 1 can French fried onions
- 1 pound chicken tenders (boneless)
- 3 tablespoons BBQ sauce
- 2 ears of corn (hulled)
- 1 tablespoon brown sugar
- 3 tablespoons chopped fresh cilantro leaves
- 1 cup canned black beans (drained and rinsed)

- 1 teaspoon paprika
- 1 teaspoon sea salt
- 1/4 cup ranch dressing
- 1/2 head of romaine lettuce (rinsed, patted dry and sliced into strips)
- 1/2 head of iceberg lettuce (rinsed, patted dry and sliced into strips)
- 1/2 teaspoon garlic powder
- 1/2 teaspoon pepper

Directions/Instructions:

1. Lightly spray each ear of corn with some oil and then place them in the cooking basket. Cook for 10 minutes at 400 degrees.

2. Mix to combine brown sugar, pepper, garlic powder, paprika, and salt in a bowl. Place the meat in the mixture and toss to coat.

3. Transfer the cooked corn to a platter and leave to cool. Cut the kernels off the cob and place them in a bowl.

4. Arrange the coated chicken tenders in the cooking basket and lightly spray with oil. Cook for 10 minutes at 400 degrees. Flip the meat halfway through the process. Transfer the cooked meat to a chopping board and dice.

5. Toss the diced meat, corn kernels and the rest of the ingredients, except for the French fried onions. Toss until combined.

6. Top with the onions before serving.

Note: You can replace chicken tenders with other meat, such as turkey, beef, or lamb. Adjust the cooking time until the meat is done.

Crispy Fried Spring Rolls

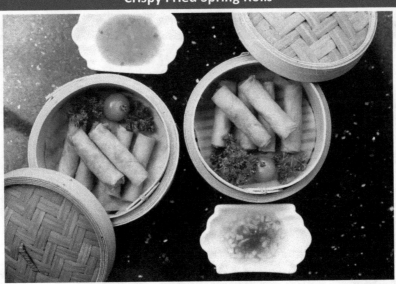

Nutritional Facts/Calories: 257 calories, 3.5g fat, 40.9g carbohydrates, 14.2g protein, 65mg cholesterol, 503mg sodium

Preparation + Cook Time: 24 minutes

Servings: 4

Ingredients:
For the filling

- 1/2 teaspoon finely chopped ginger
- 1/2 cup sliced mushrooms
- 1 teaspoon sugar
- 1 teaspoon chicken stock powder

- 4 ounces chicken breast (cooked and shredded)
- 1 carrot (thinly sliced)
- 1 celery stalk (thinly sliced)

For the spring roll wrappers

- 1/2 teaspoon vegetable oil
- 1 teaspoon cornstarch
- 8 spring roll wrappers
- 1 egg (beaten)

Directions/Instructions:

1. Prepare the filling. Put the meat, carrot, mushrooms, and celery in a bowl. Mix until combined. Add the chicken stock powder, sugar, and ginger. Mix well.

2. In another bowl, combine the cornstarch and egg and whisk until thick. Set aside.

3. Spoon some filling into a spring roll wrapper. Roll and seal the ends with the egg mixture. Brush the prepared spring rolls with a bit of oil. Arrange them in the cooking basket.

4. Cook for 4 minutes at 390 degrees.

Note: Serve the dish while warm. You can enjoy this with a variety of dipping sauces depending on your preference. You can try dipping the rolls in sweet chili sauce, vinegar or soy sauce. You can also use them as toppings of cooked rice or pasta.

Feta Triangles

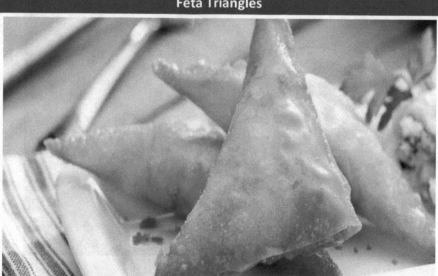

Nutritional Facts/Calories: 144 calories, 11.8g fat, 5.8g carbohydrates, 4.5g protein, 62mg cholesterol, 371mg sodium

Preparation + Cook Time: 25 minutes

Servings: 5

Ingredients:

- 2 sheets of frozen filo pastry (thawed)
- 2 tablespoons flat-leafed parsley (minced)
- Ground black pepper
- 2 tablespoons olive oil
- 4 ounces feta cheese
- 1 scallion (minced)
- 1 egg yolk

Directions/Instructions:

1. Whisk the egg yolk, scallion, parsley, and feta in a bowl until combined. Season with pepper.

2. Cut each filo sheet into 3 strips. Place a teaspoon of the feta mixture in each strip. Fold the sheet and roll all the filling is covered.

3. Lightly brush each filo with oil. Arrange 6 feta triangles in the cooking basket at a time. Cook for 3 minutes at 390 degrees. Cook for 2 more minutes at 360 degrees.

French Toast Stuffed with Blueberry Cream Cheese

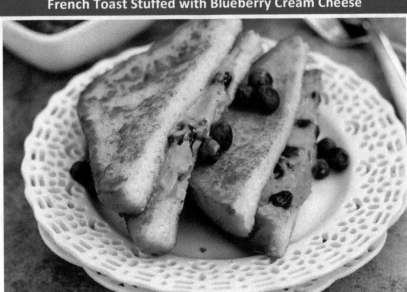

Nutritional Facts/Calories: 182 calories, 4.1g fat, 27g carbohydrates, 9.9g protein, 85mg cholesterol, 497mg sodium

Preparation + Cook Time: 18 minutes

Servings: 4

Ingredients:

- 4 tablespoons whipped cream cheese (berry-flavored)
- 2 eggs (beaten)
- 4 2-inch slices of Challah bread
- 3 teaspoons sugar
- 1/3 cup whole milk
- 1/4 cup fresh blueberries
- 1/4 teaspoon salt
- 1/4 teaspoon ground nutmeg
- 1 1/2 cups crumbled corn flakes

Directions/Instructions:

1. In a bowl, mix to combine the eggs, salt, sugar, nutmeg, and milk.

2. Put the whipped cream cheese in another bowl and fold in the blueberries.

3. Slit the top part of each Challah bread. Add 2 tablespoons of the berry mixture to each slice. Soak the stuffed bread slices in the egg mixture until completely coated. Cover them with corn flakes and gently press to make them stick.

4. Arrange the stuffed bread slices in the cooking basket of the Air Fryer. Cook for 8 minutes at 400 degrees.

Note: This is best served while warm. You can opt to drizzle it with maple syrup or add a bit of butter.

Pizza Rolls

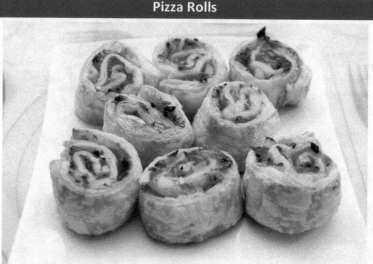

Nutritional Facts/Calories: 420 calories, 11.8g fat, 61.1g carbohydrates, 16.2g protein, 34mg cholesterol, 1013mg sodium

Preparation + Cook Time: 50 minutes

Servings: 6

Ingredients:

- 1 14-ounce jar of pizza sauce
- 2 pieces Italian sausage (cooked and crumbled)
- 1 onion (chopped)
- 15 egg roll wrappers

- 2 cups whole milk mozzarella (shredded)
- 2 red peppers (roasted and chopped)
- 3 ounces sliced pepperoni (chopped)
- 1 teaspoon garlic powder

Directions/Instructions:

1. Mix the peppers, cheese, onions, pepperoni, and sausage in a bowl. Keep on mixing as you add the garlic powder and pizza sauce.

2. Scoop 1/4 of the mixture into each egg roll wrapper. Fold all sides until the filling is wrapped. Moisten the last fold to secure. Roll it tightly. Perform the same steps with the rest of the wrappers. Put in a covered container and freeze overnight.

3. Put 5 pieces of the pizza rolls in the cooking basket at a time. Make sure that you do not overcrowd the pan because they will expand quite a lot. Lightly spray them with a non-stick cooking spray.

4. Cook for 7 minutes at 400 degrees. Flip them and continue cooking for 2 more minutes. Transfer to a platter and repeat the process with the rest of the rolls.

5. Serve the rolls with pizza sauce for dipping.

Note: You can also serve them with cheese or yogurt.

Roasted Brussels Sprouts

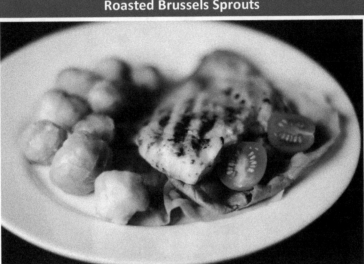

Nutritional Facts/Calories: 198 calories, 12.4g fat, 20.6g carbohydrates, 7.7g protein, 638mg sodium

Preparation + Cook Time: 20 minutes

Servings: 2

Ingredients:

- 5 teaspoons olive oil
- 1/2 teaspoon kosher salt
- 1 pound fresh Brussels sprouts

Directions/Instructions:

1. Remove outer leaves with bruises and trim the stems. Slice vertically into 2. Rinse them and shake off excess liquid. Put them in a bowl. Add olive oil and salt and toss to coat.

2. Preheat the Air Fryer at 390 degrees. Arrange the prepared sprouts in the cooking basket and cook for 15 minutes. Shake the basket occasionally during the cooking process.

Note: Although they make easy nibbles for breakfast but you can have them any time of the day. You can add more seasoning if preferred. You can use garlic powder, onion powder or cheese powder. You can also serve them along with dipping sauces.

Lunch Recipes

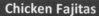

Chicken Fajitas

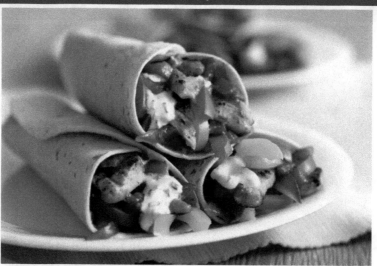

Nutritional Facts/Calories: 426 calories, 20.1g fat, 21.5g carbohydrates, 40g protein, 128mg cholesterol, 550mg sodium

Preparation + Cook Time: 34 minutes

Servings: 4

Ingredients:

- 4 flour tortillas (premade)
- 1/2 teaspoon sea salt
- 1/2 teaspoon chili powder
- 1/4 teaspoon ground coriander
- 1/4 teaspoon ground cumin
- 1/4 teaspoon ground black pepper

For garnishing

- 1 cup lettuce (shredded)
- 1/2 cup medium salsa

- 1 pound chicken breasts (cut into strips)
- 1 onion (peeled and chopped)
- 1 green pepper (cored and sliced)
- 1 red pepper (cored and sliced)
- 1 tablespoon fresh lime juice
- 1 teaspoon garlic powder

- 1/2 cup sour cream
- 1/2 cup shredded cheddar cheese

Directions/Instructions:

1. In a bowl, put the coriander, garlic powder, salt, cumin, chili powder, and pepper. Mix well. Add the meat and lime juice. Stir and leave to marinate for 10 minutes. Add the peppers and onion, and toss to combine.

2. Put half of the mixture in the cooking basket of the Air Fryer. Spray it with non-stick cooking spray. Set the fryer to 400 degrees and cook for 8 minutes. Transfer to a platter and cook the remaining mixture.

3. Put the tortillas in the cooking basket. Set the fryer to 190 degrees and cook for 3 minutes.

4. Divide the cooked meat as filling for the tortillas. Serve with the ingredients for garnishing.

Chicken Nuggets

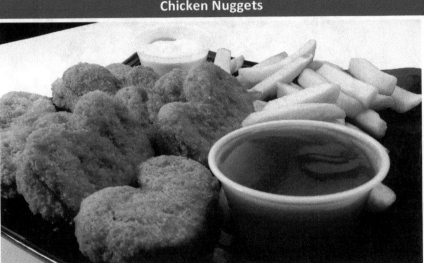

Nutritional Facts/Calories: 356 calories, 9.3g fat, 27.2g carbohydrates, 38.2g protein, 103mg cholesterol, 744mg sodium

Preparation + Cook Time: 45 minutes

Servings: 4

Ingredients:

- 1 cup buttermilk
- 1 teaspoon salt
- 1/2 teaspoon garlic powder
- 1/2 teaspoon paprika
- 1 pound chicken breasts (skinless and boneless, chopped)
- 1 cup flour

Directions/Instructions:

1. Place meat in a bowl and cover with buttermilk. Leave for an hour or overnight to marinate.

2. In a bowl, mix flour, garlic powder, paprika, and salt until well combined. Add the meat and toss until coated. Arrange 8 chicken nuggets in the cooking basket at a time. Lightly spray them with oil.

3. Cook for 10 minutes at 400 degrees.

4. Transfer to a platter and cook the remaining nuggets.

Note: Serve the dish with a variety of sauces for dipping.

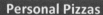

Personal Pizzas

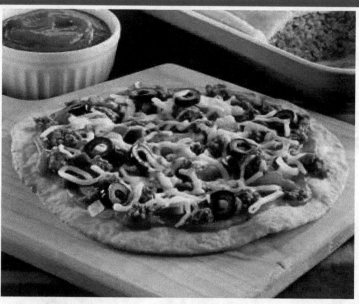

Nutritional Facts/Calories: 207 calories, 10.4g fat, 23.1g carbohydrates, 6.7g protein, 6mg cholesterol, 540mg sodium

Preparation + Cook Time: 45 minutes

Servings: 2

Ingredients:

- 1/2 cup of mozzarella cheese (shredded)
- 1/4 cup of Parmesan cheese (grated)
- A pinch of garlic powder
- A pinch of dried oregano
- 1 can of pizza crust

- 1 tablespoon olive oil
- 1/2 cup pizza sauce (store-bought or homemade)
- Toppings of your choice

Directions/Instructions:

1. Cut the dough into 4 and roll each piece into a ball. Rub them with olive oil and stretch each dough ball in a pizza pan.

2. Spread 1/4 of the sauce to each stretched dough in the pan. Add 1 tablespoon of parmesan, 2 tablespoons of mozzarella cheese, a pinch of garlic powder and a pinch of dried oregano on top. Add your preferred toppings.

3. Place a rack in the cooking basket and put the pizza pan on top of it. Cook for 6 minutes at 350 degrees.

4. Transfer to a plate and slice into 4.

5. Repeat the steps to cook the remaining dough.

Note: Adjust the nutri info depending on the toppings used. You can try adding different toppings depending on your preference. You can use pepperoni, ham, mushrooms, pineapple, crumbled sausage, meatballs, peppers, and many more.

Portabella Pepperoni Pizza

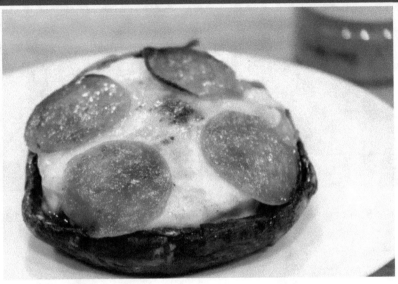

Nutritional Facts/Calories: 320 calories, 28.8g fat, 3.3g carbohydrates, 13.9g protein, 38mg cholesterol, 666mg sodium

Preparation + Cook Time: 11 minutes

Servings: 3

Ingredients:

- 12 pepperoni slices
- 3 tablespoons shredded mozzarella cheese
- 3 tablespoons tomato sauce
- 3 tablespoons olive oil
- 3 portabella mushroom caps (rinsed and scooped)
- A pinch of dried Italian seasonings
- A pinch of salt

Directions/Instructions:

1. Pour a bit of oil on both sides of the mushroom caps. Season the inner part with Italian seasonings and salt. Drizzle tomato sauce on top and add cheese. Arrange them in the cooking basket. Cook for 1 minute at 330 degrees.

2. Add pepperoni slices on top of each portabella and continue cooking for 5 more minutes.

3. Transfer to a plate and serve while warm.

Note: You can sprinkle more cheese while the dish is still hot. You can also opt to sprinkle them with crushed red pepper flakes.

Dinner Recipes

Barbeque Chicken

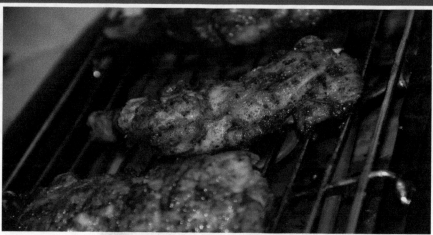

Nutritional Facts/Calories: 356 calories, 11g fat, 19.4g carbohydrates, 42.7g protein, 130mg cholesterol, 798mg sodium

Preparation + Cook Time: 40 minutes

Servings: 2

Ingredients:

- 1 tablespoon molasses
- 1 tablespoon cider vinegar
- 1 tablespoon ketchup
- 2 tablespoons brown sugar
- 2 chicken thighs

- 1/4 teaspoon paprika
- 1/4 teaspoon dry mustard
- 1/2 teaspoon garlic powder
- 1/2 teaspoon salt
- 1/2 teaspoon freshly ground pepper

Directions/Instructions:

1. Put all the ingredients, except the meat in a bowl. Mix well. Soak the meat into the mixture and leave for 30 minutes to marinate.

2. Place the rack in the cooking basket and put the meat on top. Baste the meat with the remaining marinade. Cook for 15 minutes at 380 degrees. Flip the meat, baste with the marinade and cook for 10 more minutes.

Chicken Buffalo Drummies

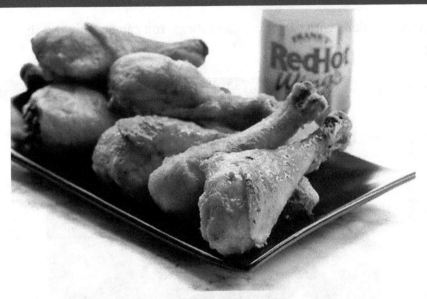

Nutritional Facts/Calories: 1927 calories, 76.3g fat, 90.2g carbohydrates, 207.9g protein, 684mg cholesterol, 15862mg sodium

Preparation + Cook Time: 40 minutes

Servings: 2

Ingredients:

- 10 chicken drummies (bone-in)
- 1 cup rice flour
- 3 cups water
- 1 cup ice

For the buffalo sauce

- 1 teaspoon soy sauce
- 1 teaspoon cider vinegar
- 1 teaspoon ketchup

- 1 teaspoon cayenne
- 1/4 cup sugar
- 1/4 cup salt

- 4 tablespoons hot sauce
- 4 tablespoons melted unsalted butter

Directions/Instructions:

1. Put water, sugar, and salt in a stainless container. Stir until dissolved. Stir in the cayenne pepper. Add the meat and put ice on top. Leave for 2 to 12 hours to brine.

2. Mix to combine all the ingredients for the sauce in a bowl.

3. Remove the meat from the brine mixture and pat them dry. Coat with rice flour and arrange in the cooking basket.

4. Cook for 25 minutes at 400 degrees. Shake the cooking basket twice during the cooking process.

5. Put sauce in a bowl. Add the cooked meat and toss until coated.

Note: You can serve this dish along with carrot or celery sticks. You can also dip the chicken wings on a ranch or blue cheese dressing.

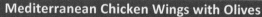

Mediterranean Chicken Wings with Olives

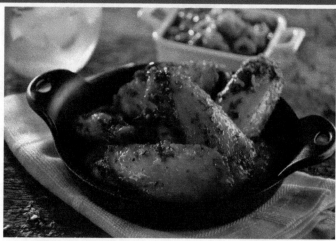

Nutritional Facts/Calories: 344 calories, 14.5g fat, 1.4g carbohydrates, 49.4g protein, 151mg cholesterol, 332mg sodium

Preparation + Cook Time: 40 minutes

Servings: 4

Ingredients:

- 1/2 cup olives
- 1 1/2 pounds chicken wings
- 1 teaspoon oregano
- 1 1/2 teaspoons lemon juice
- A pinch of salt
- A pinch of garlic powder

Directions/Instructions:

1. Mix to combine salt, lemon juice, garlic powder, and oregano in a bowl. Add the meat and toss until coated.

2. Arrange half of the seasoned meat in the cooking basket. Cook for 10 minutes at 356 degrees. Shake the basket twice during the process. Add the olives and cook for 5 more minutes. Perform the same cooking process with the remaining chicken wings.

3. Serve while hot.

Roasted Rack of Lamb with Macadamia Crust

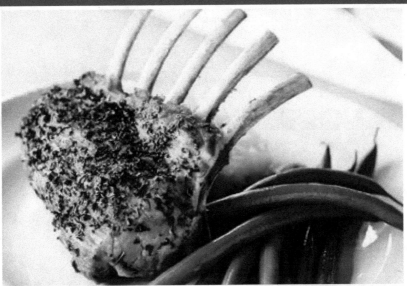

Nutritional Facts/Calories: 215 calories, 16.9g fat, 3.4g carbohydrates, 13.7g protein, 64mg cholesterol, 51mg sodium

Preparation + Cook Time: 45 minutes

Servings: 6

Ingredients:

- 1 3/4 pound rack of lamb
- 1 garlic clove (peeled and minced)
- Salt and pepper to taste
- 1 tablespoon olive oil

For the macadamia crust

- 3 ounces macadamia nuts (finely chopped)
- 1 tablespoon breadcrumbs
- 1 tablespoon fresh rosemary (chopped)
- 1 egg

Directions/Instructions:

1. Prepare garlic oil. Put olive oil and minced garlic in a bowl and mix well.

2. Brush the meat with garlic oil. Season with salt and pepper.

3. Put the chopped nuts, rosemary, and breadcrumbs in a bowl. Mix well.

4. Whisk the eggs in another bowl.

5. Dip the lamb into the egg mixture. Drain the excess liquid and cover with the macadamia crust. Arrange the coated meat in the cooking basket.

6. Cook for 30 minutes at 220 degrees. Cook for 5 more minutes at 390 degrees.

7. Transfer into a plate and loosely cover with a foil. Leave for 10 minutes to rest before serving.

Poultry Recipes

Buffalo Chicken Tenders

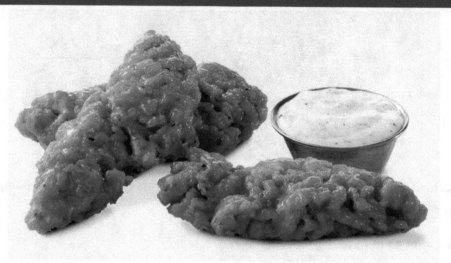

Nutritional Facts/Calories: 380 calories, 12.1g fat, 28g carbohydrates, 41g protein, 110mg cholesterol, 850mg sodium

Preparation + Cook Time: 34 minutes

Servings: 4

Ingredients:

- 1/2 cup Buffalo sauce
- 1 cup flour
- 1 pound chicken tenders (trimmed)
- 1 cup ranch dressing
- 1/4 cup blue cheese (crumbled)
- 1/2 teaspoon garlic powder
- 1/2 teaspoon cayenne pepper
- 1/2 teaspoon salt

Directions/Instructions:

1. Put the ranch dressing in a bowl. Add the meat and leave to marinate for an hour.

2. Mix to combine flour, cayenne pepper, salt, and garlic powder in a bowl. Dip each chicken piece in the mixture until coated. Put 2 chicken tenders in the cooking basket at a time

3. Cook for 13 minutes at 400 degrees. Shake the basket twice during the cooking process. Transfer the cooked meat to a bowl and cook the rest.

4. Put the buffalo sauce in a bowl. Add the cooked meat and toss until coated. Transfer to a plate and sprinkle with cheese before serving.

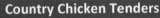

Country Chicken Tenders

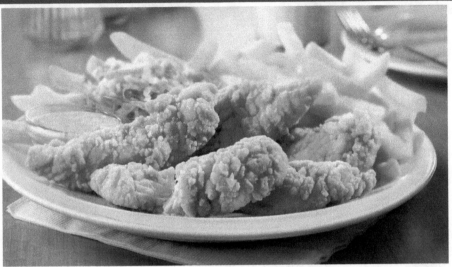

Nutritional Facts/Calories: 486 calories, 21.6g fat, 29.5g carbohydrates, 41g protein, 210mg cholesterol, 659mg sodium

Preparation + Cook Time: 30 minutes

Servings: 3

Ingredients:

- 3/4 pound chicken tenders

For the breading

- 1/2 cup seasoned breadcrumbs
- 2 tablespoons olive oil
- 2 eggs (beaten)

- 1 teaspoon black pepper
- 1/2 teaspoon salt
- 1/2 cup all-purpose flour

Directions/Instructions:

1. Combine breadcrumbs and salt in a bowl. Add olive oil and mix well.

2. Put the beaten eggs in a different bowl and flour in another.

3. Toss meat in the bowl of flour until coated. Dip them in egg and coat with the breadcrumb mixture. Press using your hands to make the coating stick to the meat. Arrange them in the cooking basket.

4. Cook for 10 minutes at 330 degrees. Turn the temperature to 350 degrees and cook for 5 more minutes.

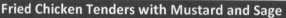

Fried Chicken Tenders with Mustard and Sage

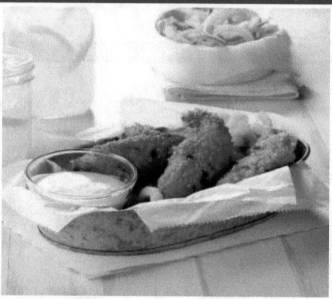

Nutritional Facts/Calories: 727 calories, 30.9g fat, 21.6g carbohydrates, 85g protein, 266mg cholesterol, 532mg sodium

Preparation + Cook Time: 30 minutes

Servings: 2

Ingredients:

- 1 tablespoon melted butter
- 1 tablespoon mayonnaise
- 1/2 cup panko breadcrumbs

- 1/2 teaspoon dry sage
- 4 chicken tenders
- 1 teaspoon Dijon mustard

Directions/Instructions:

1. Mix to combine sage, mustard, and mayonnaise in a bowl.

2. In another bowl, put the butter and breadcrumbs and mix well.

3. Pat the meat dry using paper towels. Coat each piece with a bit of the mayonnaise mixture and cover with the breadcrumb mixture.

4. Arrange in a single layer in the cooking basket. Cook for 10 minutes at 392 degrees. Flip the meat and cook for 10 more minutes.

Jerk Chicken Wings

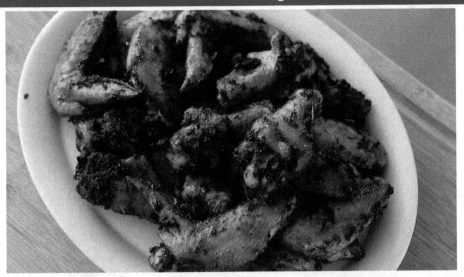

Nutritional Facts/Calories: 623 calories, 27.8g fat, 13.6g carbohydrates, 801g protein, 242mg cholesterol, 1050mg sodium

Preparation + Cook Time: 33 minutes

Servings: 5

Ingredients:

- 5 tablespoons lime juice
- 1 habanero pepper (remove the ribs and seeds, chopped)
- 1/2 cup red wine vinegar
- 3 pounds chicken wings
- 6 garlic cloves (minced)
- 2 tablespoons soy sauce
- 2 tablespoons olive oil
- 1 teaspoon white pepper

- 1 teaspoon salt
- 1 teaspoon cinnamon
- 1 teaspoon cayenne pepper
- 1 tablespoon grated fresh ginger
- 1 tablespoon chopped fresh thyme
- 1 tablespoon allspice
- 2 tablespoons brown sugar
- 4 scallions (minced)

Directions/Instructions:

1. Put all ingredients in a bowl and mix until combined and the meat is well-coated. Transfer to a Ziploc bag. Refrigerate for 2 hours or overnight.

2. Drain the liquid and pat the meat dry using paper towels. Arrange them in the cooking basket.

3. Cook for 18 minutes at 390 degrees. Shake the basket halfway through the cooking process.

Note: Serve the dish along with your favorite sauces. You can also try it with ranch dressing or blue cheese dipping sauce.

Korean BBQ Satay

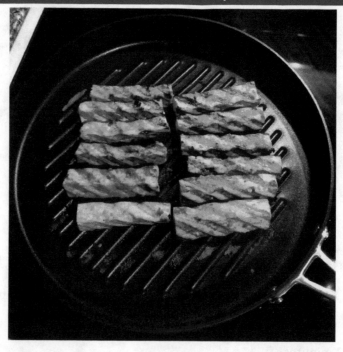

Nutritional Facts/Calories: 442 calories, 27.8g fat, 12.6g carbohydrates, 41g protein, 110mg cholesterol, 2450mg sodium

Preparation + Cook Time: 22 minutes

Servings: 3

Ingredients:

- 1 tablespoon grated fresh ginger
- 2 teaspoons toasted sesame seeds
- 1/2 cup pineapple juice
- 1/2 cup low-sodium soy sauce
- 1/4 cup sesame oil

- 4 garlic cloves (chopped)
- 12 ounces chicken tenders (boneless and skinless)
- 4 scallions (chopped)
- A pinch of black pepper

Directions/Instructions:

1. Skewer each piece of meat and trim excess fat.

2. Put the remaining ingredients in a bowl. Mix well. Add the skewered chicken and make sure that all pieces are covered with the mixture. Cover the bowl and refrigerate for 2 hours or overnight.

3. Use paper towels to pat the meat dry. Arrange the skewers in the cooking basket. Cook for 7 minutes at 390 degrees.

Pork Recipes

Asian Style Baby Back Ribs

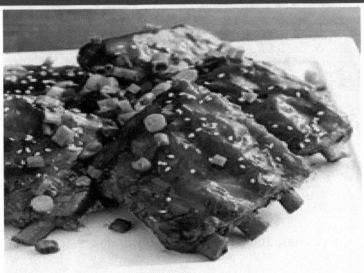

Nutritional Facts/Calories: 346 calories, 27g fat, 15g carbohydrates, 9.1g protein, 48mg cholesterol, 45mg sodium

Preparation + Cook Time: 1 hour 15 minutes

Servings: 2

Ingredients:

- 2 tablespoons sesame oil
- 1 jalapeño (seeded and chopped)
- 1/2 tablespoon chopped cilantro
- 1 slab baby back ribs

- 1 scallion (finely chopped)
- 1 cup orange juice
- 1 teaspoon grated ginger
- 1 garlic clove (minced)

Directions/Instructions:

1. Put all the ingredients in a Ziploc bag and seal. Shake until all sides of the meat are coated. Refrigerate overnight to marinate.

2. Reserve the marinade. Arrange the ribs in the cooking basket in a vertical position. Cook for 35 minutes at 350 degrees.

3. Pour the marinade in a pan over medium-high flame. Cook until the liquid is reduced by half. Turn off the stove.

4. Brush the half-cooked ribs with the marinade and cook for 30 more minutes.

5. Transfer to a plate and slice. Serve along with the remaining marinade.

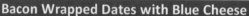

Bacon Wrapped Dates with Blue Cheese

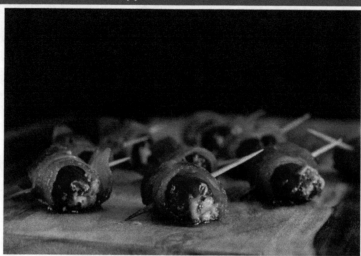

Nutritional Facts/Calories: 174 calories, 10.8g fat, 11g carbohydrates, 9.1g protein, 28mg cholesterol, 565mg sodium

Preparation + Cook Time: 28 minutes

Servings: 6

Ingredients:

- 1 teaspoon Cajun seasoning
- 1/4 pound blue cheese (cut into 10)
- 10 Medjool dates (pitted)
- 4 bacon strips (cut into 3)

Directions/Instructions:

1. Insert blue cheese inside each date. Wrap the filled dates with bacon. Secure its hold with a toothpick. Arrange them in the cooking basket.

2. Cook for 5 minutes at 400 degrees. Flip the dates and cook for 3 more minutes.

3. Transfer to a platter and sprinkle with Cajun seasoning before serving.

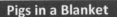

Pigs in a Blanket

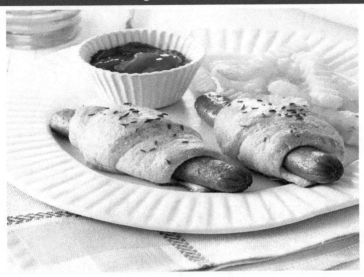

Nutritional Facts/Calories: 513 calories, 34.5g fat, 31.8g carbohydrates, 17.9g protein, 63mg cholesterol, 989mg sodium

Preparation + Cook Time: 31 minutes

Servings: 4

Ingredients:

- 1 8-ounce can of crescent rolls
- 1 12-ounce package of cocktail franks

Directions/Instructions:

1. Drain the liquid from the cocktail franks. Use paper towels to pat them dry.

2. Cut the dough into strips. Roll each strip into a piece of the frank. Leave the edges visible. Chill for 5 minutes or until firm.

3. Arrange the wrapped cocktail franks in the cooking basket. Cook for 8 minutes at 330 degrees. Turn the temperature setting to 390 degrees and cook for 3 more minutes.

Pizza Rolls

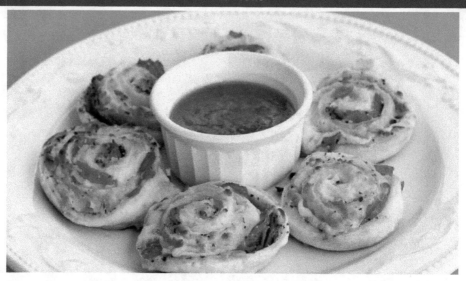

Nutritional Facts/Calories: 170 calories, 10g fat, 12.9g carbohydrates, 9g protein, 26mg cholesterol, 5801mg sodium

Preparation + Cook Time: 50 minutes

Servings: 6

Ingredients:

- 1 14-ounce jar of pizza sauce
- 2 pieces of Italian sausage (cooked and crumbled)
- 1 onion (chopped)
- 15 eggroll wrappers

- 2 cups shredded mozzarella cheese
- 2 red peppers (roasted and chopped)
- 3 ounces sliced pepperoni (chopped)
- 1 teaspoon garlic powder

Directions/Instructions:

1. Mix to combine the peppers, cheese, onions, pepperoni, and sausage in a bowl. Add the garlic powder and pizza sauce. Mix well. Scoop 1/4 of the mixture to each eggroll wrapper. Fold all sides until the filling is wrapped. Moisten the last fold to secure. Roll it tightly. Perform the same steps with the rest of the wrappers. Put in a container, cover and freeze overnight.

2. Arrange 5 rolls in the cooking basket at a time and lightly spray them with a non-stick cooking spray. Cook for 7 minutes at 400 degrees and cook for 7 minutes. Flip the pizza rolls and cook for 2 more minutes. Transfer to a platter and cook the remaining rolls.

3. Serve the rolls with pizza sauce for dipping.

Beef Recipes

Chimichurri Skirt Steak

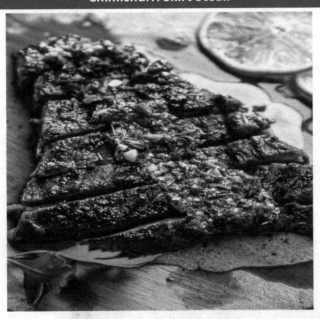

Nutritional Facts/Calories: 1175 calories, 100.3g fat, 10.6g carbohydrates, 61g protein, 134mg cholesterol, 1570mg sodium

Preparation + Cook Time: 25 minutes

Servings: 2

Ingredients:

- 1 pound skirt steak

For the chimichurri

- 3 garlic cloves (minced)
- 1/4 cup finely chopped mint
- 1 tablespoon ground cumin
- 3/4 cup olive oil
- 1/4 teaspoon black pepper
- 2 tablespoons minced oregano
- 1 cup chopped parsley
- 1 teaspoon cayenne pepper
- 1 teaspoon crushed red pepper
- 1 teaspoon salt
- 3 tablespoons red wine vinegar
- 2 teaspoons smoked paprika

Directions/Instructions:

1. Put all the ingredients for the chimichurri in a bowl. Mix well. Pour 1/4 cup of the mixture to a Ziploc bag.

2. Slice the steak into 2. Put them in a Ziploc bag along with the chimichurri. Seal the bag and shake until all sides of the meat are coated. Refrigerate for at least 2 hours or overnight.

3. Leave the marinated meat at room temperature half an hour before cooking. Drain the liquid and pat the meat with paper towels to dry.

4. Arrange the meat in the cooking basket. Cook for 10 minutes at 390 degrees for a medium-rare steak. Add more minutes if you want it well done.

5. Transfer to a platter and drizzle with 2 tablespoons of chimichurri before serving.

Fried Meatballs in Tomato Sauce

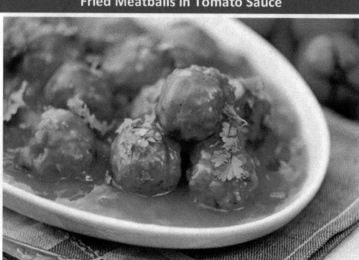

Nutritional Facts/Calories: 436 calories, 14g fat, 10.8g carbohydrates, 63.6g protein, 218mg cholesterol, 557mg sodium

Preparation + Cook Time: 25 minutes

Servings: 4

Ingredients:

- 3/4 pound ground beef
- Salt and pepper to taste
- 1 tablespoon chopped parsley
- 1/2 tablespoon fresh thyme leaves (chopped)

- 10 ounces tomato sauce
- 1 egg
- 1 onion (chopped)
- 3 tablespoons breadcrumbs

Directions/Instructions:

1. Put all the ingredients in a bowl and mix until combined. Use your hands to form 12 small balls from the mixture. Arrange them in the cooking basket.

2. Cook for 8 minutes at 390 degrees. Transfer the meatballs to an oven dish. Drizzle with tomato sauce on top.

3. Place the oven dish in the cooking basket and cook for 5 minutes at 330 degrees.

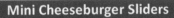

Mini Cheeseburger Sliders

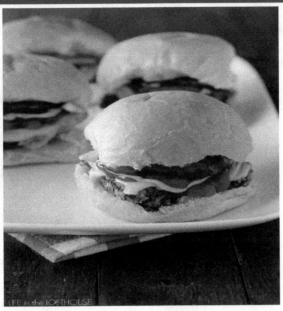

Nutritional Facts/Calories: 555 calories, 28g fat, 9.1g carbohydrates, 61g protein, 194mg cholesterol, 570mg sodium

Preparation + Cook Time: 19 minutes

Servings: 3

Ingredients:

- 6 slices of cheddar cheese
- Salt and black pepper to taste
- 1 pound ground beef
- 6 dinner rolls

Directions/Instructions:

1. Divide the meat into 6 and form them into patties. Season with salt and pepper.

2. Arrange the patties in the cooking basket. Cook for 10 minutes at 390 degrees. Place cheese on top of each patty and continue cooking for a minute.

3. Fill each dinner roll with the cooked patty.

Seafood Recipes

Bacon Wrapped Shrimp

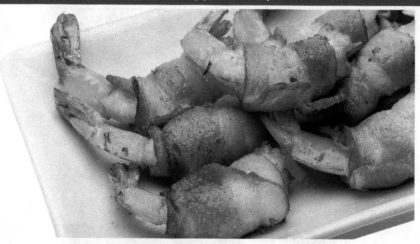

Nutritional Facts/Calories: 436 calories, 41.01g fat, 0.86g carbohydrates, 15.64g protein, 32mg cholesterol, 600mg sodium

Preparation + Cook Time: 32 minutes

Servings: 4

Ingredients:

- 16 thin slices of bacon
- 16 pieces of tiger shrimp (peeled and deveined)

Directions/Instructions:

1. Wrap each shrimp with a slice of bacon. Put all the finished pieces in tray and chill for 20 minutes.

2. Arrange the bacon wrapped shrimp in the cooking basket. Cook for 7 minutes at 390 degrees. Transfer to a plate lined with paper towels to drain before serving.

Cod Fish Nuggets

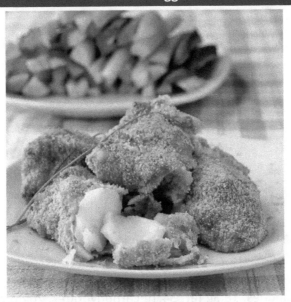

Nutritional Facts/Calories: 404 calories, 11.6g fat, 38.6g carbohydrates, 34.6g protein, 144mg cholesterol, 307mg sodium

Preparation + Cook Time: 25 minutes

Servings: 4

Ingredients:

- 1 pound of cod (cut into strips)

For the breading

- 2 eggs (beaten)
- 3/4 cup breadcrumbs
- 1 cup all-purpose flour
- 2 tablespoons olive oil
- A pinch of salt

Directions/Instructions:

1. Put olive oil, salt, and panko breadcrumbs in a food processor. Process until fine. Transfer mixture to a bowl.

2. Put the flour and the beaten eggs in separate bowls.

3. Coat each cod strip with flour. Dip in the eggs and coat with breadcrumbs. Press the coating to make it stick.

4. Arrange the coated cod pieces in the cooking basket. Cook for 10 minutes at 390 degrees.

Crab Croquettes

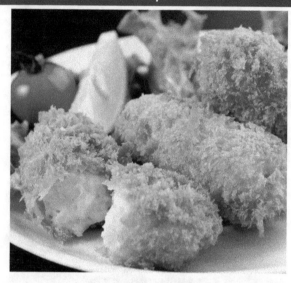

Nutritional Facts/Calories: 322 calories, 18.3g fat, 34.1g carbohydrates, 20g protein, 131mg cholesterol, 872mg sodium

Preparation + Cook Time: 30 minutes

Servings: 6

Ingredients:

- 1/4 cup red onion (finely chopped)
- 1/4 cup sour cream
- 1/4 cup mayonnaise
- 1/2 teaspoon cayenne pepper
- 1/2 teaspoon parsley (finely chopped)
- 1 tablespoon olive oil

- 2 tablespoons celery (finely chopped)
- 2 egg whites (beaten)
- 1 pound of lump crab meat
- 1/4 red bell pepper (chopped)
- 1/4 teaspoon chives (finely chopped)
- 1/4 teaspoon tarragon

For the breading

- 3 eggs (beaten)
- 1 teaspoon olive oil
- 1 cup panko breadcrumbs

- 1 cup all-purpose flour
- 1/2 teaspoon salt

Directions/Instructions:

1. Heat oil in a pan over medium-high flame. Add the onions, celery, and peppers. Saute for 5 minutes. Remove from heat and set aside.

2. Put the breadcrumbs, salt, and olive oil in a food processor. Process until fine.

3. Put the flour, panko mixture, and eggs in 3 separate bowls.

4. Put the crabmeat, mayonnaise, egg whites, spices, vegetables, and sour cream in a bowl and mix until combined. Use your hands to shape them into golf-size crabmeat balls.

5. Roll each ball into the flour, eggs, and panko mixture. Press the coating to make them stick.

6. Arrange them in the cooking basket. Cook for 10 minutes at 390 degrees.

Fish Tacos

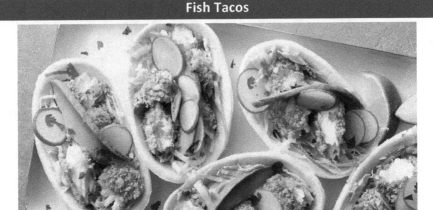

Nutritional Facts/Calories: 618 calories, 17g fat, 71.7g carbohydrates, 36g protein, 104mg cholesterol, 1381mg sodium

Preparation + Cook Time: 17 minutes

Servings: 4

Ingredients:

- 2 snapper or grouper fillets
- 1 egg
- 1 cup plain breadcrumbs
- 1 cup panko breadcrumbs
- 6 taco shells (premade)
- 1 cup salsa
- 1 cup shredded lettuce
- 1 cup, plus 1/2 cup of sour cream
- 1/2 cup medium salsa
- 1/2 cup shredded low-fat cheddar cheese
- 1/2 cup buttermilk
- 1/4 cup flour
- 1/4 teaspoon black pepper
- 1/2 teaspoon garlic powder
- 1/2 teaspoon salt

Directions/Instructions:

1. Put the flour, egg, and buttermilk in a bowl. Mix well until combined. Set aside.

2. Put the breadcrumbs, black pepper, salt, and garlic powder in a shallow dish and mix well.

3. Dip the fillets in the egg mixture and coat each piece with the breadcrumbs mixture.

4. Arrange the coated fillets in the cooking basket and lightly spray with oil. Cook for 12 minutes at 400 degrees.

5. Put cheese, sour cream, salsa, and lettuce in taco shells and top with the cooked fillets.

Fish with Chips

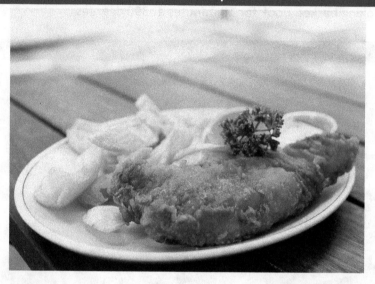

Nutritional Facts/Calories: 646 calories, 33g fat, 48g carbohydrates, 41g protein, 94mg cholesterol, 1781mg sodium

Preparation + Cook Time: 22 minutes

Servings: 2

Ingredients:

- 1 cod fillet (6 ounces)
- 3 cups salt
- 3 cups vinegar-flavored kettle cooked chips
- 1/4 cup buttermilk
- 1/4 teaspoon pepper
- 1/2 teaspoon salt

Directions/Instructions:

1. Mix to combine the buttermilk, pepper, and salt in a bowl. Put the cod and leave to soak for 5 minutes.

2. Put the chips in a food processor and process until crushed. Transfer to a shallow bowl. Coat the fillet with the crushed chips.

3. Put the coated fillet in the cooking basket. Cook for 12 minutes at 400 degrees.

Salmon with Dill Sauce

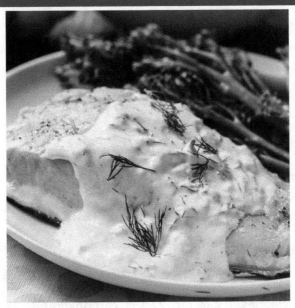

Nutritional Facts/Calories: 348 calories, 18.97g fat, 5.29g carbohydrates, 37.694g protein, 128mg cholesterol, 814mg sodium

Preparation + Cook Time: 45 minutes

Servings: 4

Ingredients:

- 2 teaspoons olive oil
- 4 6-ounce pieces of salmon

For the dill sauce

- 1/2 cup sour cream
- 1/2 cup Greek yogurt (non-fat)

- A pinch of salt

- 2 tablespoons finely chopped dill
- A pinch of salt

Directions/Instructions:

1. Drizzle each piece of salmon with olive oil. Season with salt. Put them in the cooking basket. Cook for 30 minutes at 270 degrees.

2. Prepare the sauce. Combine all the ingredients for the sauce in a bowl. Mix well.

3. Serve the fish with the sauce. Top with chopped dill.

Tuna Melt Sandwich

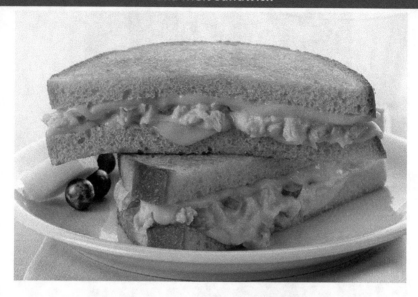

Nutritional Facts/Calories: 261 calories, 8.43g fat, 27.15g carbohydrates, 22.46g protein, 32mg cholesterol, 583mg sodium

Preparation + Cook Time: 21 minutes

Servings: 2

Ingredients:

- 1 celery stalk (finely chopped)
- 1/2 cup shredded sharp cheddar cheese
- 1/8 teaspoon celery salt
- 1 teaspoon onion (finely chopped)
- A pinch of black pepper

- 1 5-ounce can of solid white tuna in water (drained)
- 2 slices of bread (multi-grain)
- 2 tablespoons mayonnaise
- 4 slices of ripe tomato

Directions/Instructions:

1. Put the bread slices in the cooking basket. Cook for 3 minutes at 400 degrees.

2. In a bowl, mix to combine the mayonnaise, tuna, salt, pepper, onion, and celery. Spread the mixture in the 2 toasted bread slices. Add 2 tomato slices and cheese on top of each bread slice.

3. Put one sandwich in the cooking basket at a time. Cook for 4 minutes at 400 degrees. Repeat the same step with the other sandwich

Vegetable Recipes

Asparagus Frittata

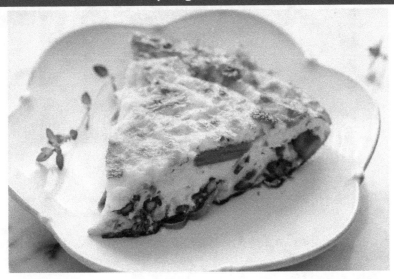

Nutritional Facts/Calories: 320 calories, 21.59g fat, 9.1g carbohydrates, 21.59g protein, 1245mg cholesterol, 311mg sodium

Preparation + Cook Time: 20 minutes

Servings: 1

Ingredients:

- 2 tablespoons milk
- 2 eggs
- Salt and pepper to taste

- 1 tablespoon Parmesan cheese (freshly grated)
- 5 asparagus tips (steamed)

Directions/Instructions:

1. Whisk the eggs, milk, salt, pepper, and cheese in a bowl until combined. Transfer to a greased baking dish. Put the steamed asparagus on top.

2. Place the rack inside the cooking basket and put the baking dish on top. Cook for 5 minutes at 400 degrees.

Crusty Potato Wedges

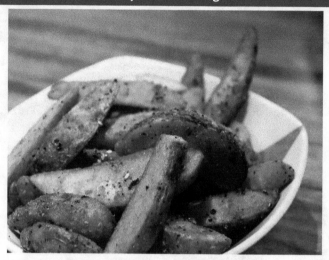

Nutritional Facts/Calories: 207 calories, 4.39g fat, 34.71g carbohydrates, 8.05g protein, 160mg cholesterol, 441mg sodium

Preparation + Cook Time: 35 minutes

Servings: 4

Ingredients:

- 1 teaspoon dried thyme
- 1 teaspoon garlic powder
- 1/4 cup grated Parmesan cheese
- 1/2 tablespoon dried rosemary
- 2 potatoes (sliced into wedges)

- 1/2 teaspoon paprika
- 1/2 teaspoon salt
- 1/2 teaspoon pepper
- 1 egg (beaten)

Directions/Instructions:

1. In a bowl, mix to combine the Parmesan cheese, rosemary, garlic powder, salt, pepper, thyme, and paprika.

2. Dip the potato wedges in the beaten egg. Put them in the spiced cheese mixture and toss until coated.

3. Arrange the coated potato wedges in the cooking basket. Lightly spray them with oil. Cook for 20 minutes at 400 degrees. Shake the basket twice during the cooking duration.

Fried Green Tomatoes

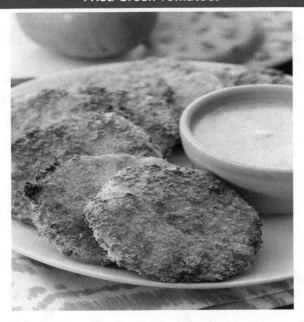

Nutritional Facts/Calories: 249 calories, 2.24g fat, 46.95g carbohydrates, 10.63g protein, 5mg cholesterol, 1654mg sodium

Preparation + Cook Time: 25 minutes

Servings: 2

Ingredients:

- 1 teaspoon salt
- 1/2 tablespoon Creole seasoning
- 1/2 teaspoon pepper
- 2 green tomatoes
- 1 cup buttermilk
- 1 cup panko breadcrumbs
- 1/2 cup instant flour

Directions/Instructions:

1. Slice the tomatoes to 1/4-inch thickness. Season both sides with salt and pepper.

2. Put the buttermilk and flour in 2 different bowls.

3. Mix the Creole seasoning and panko crumbs in another bowl.

4. Dredge each slice of tomato in the flour. Soak it in the buttermilk and coat with the panko mixture. Gently press the coating using your hands to make them stick.

5. Put the rack in the cooking basket and arrange 3 coated tomato slices on top of the rack. Lightly spray them with oil. Cook for 5 minutes at 400 degrees. Transfer to a plate and cook the remaining tomato slices.

6. Sprinkle the cooked tomatoes with your preferred amount of Creole seasoning.

Note: You can serve the dish along with a ranch dressing.

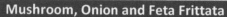

Mushroom, Onion and Feta Frittata

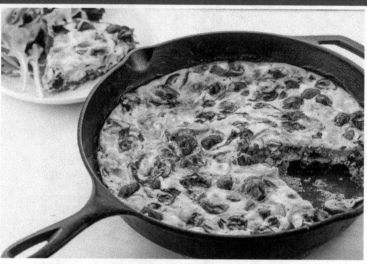

Nutritional Facts/Calories: 352 calories, 26.42g fat, 9.22g carbohydrates, 20.47g protein, 941mg cholesterol, 570mg sodium

Preparation + Cook Time: 29 minutes

Servings: 4

Ingredients:

- 4 cups button mushrooms (rinsed and thinly sliced)
- 2 tablespoons olive oil
- 1 red onion (peeled and thinly sliced)
- 6 tablespoons crumbled feta cheese
- 6 eggs
- A pinch of salt

Directions/Instructions:

1. Heat oil in a pan over medium flame. Cook the onions and mushrooms for 3 minutes. Transfer to a bowl and set aside.

2. Whisk the eggs and a pinch of salt in a bowl. Transfer to a lightly greased baking dish. Add the cooked mushroom, onion, and cheese.

3. Place the rack in the cooking basket and put the baking dish on top. Cook for 30 minutes at 330 degrees.

Noodley Kebabs

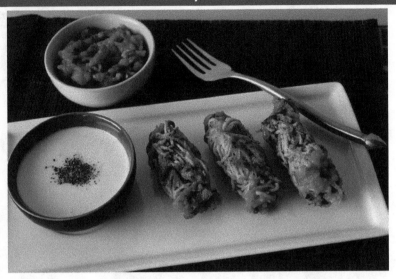

Nutritional Facts/Calories: 383 calories, 28.16g fat, 31.65g carbohydrates, 4.12g protein, 213mg sodium

Preparation + Cook Time: 1 hour 10 minutes

Servings: 4

Ingredients:

- 2 bread slices (turned into breadcrumbs)
- 1/2 teaspoon soy sauce
- 1 tablespoon coriander (chopped)
- 2 potatoes (boiled and grated)
- 1 onion

- 1/2 cup mixed vegetables (partially boiled)
- 2 teaspoons chopped ginger
- 2 green chilies
- Red chili powder to taste
- Salt to taste

For Coating

- 3/4 cup noodles (boiled)
- Milk

Directions/Instructions:

1. In a bowl, mix to combine mixed veggies, grated potatoes, salt, green chilies, soy sauce, and ginger. Use your hands to shape the mixture into small oval croquettes.

2. Dip each croquette in milk and wrap with the boiled noodles.

2. Arrange them in the cooking basket. Cook for 30 minutes at 350 degrees. Flip them halfway through the cooking process.

3. Serve while hot with tomato sauce on the side.

Stuffed Garlic Mushrooms

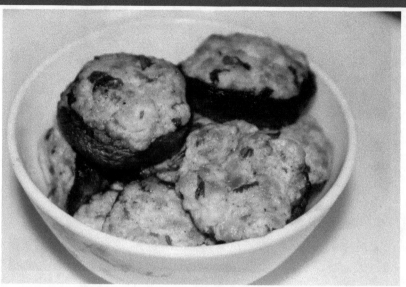

Nutritional Facts/Calories: 89 calories, 5.58g fat, 7.63g carbohydrates, 3.48g protein, 55mg sodium

Preparation + Cook Time: 23 minutes

Servings: 4

Ingredients:

- 16 button mushrooms

For the stuffing

- 1 1/2 slices of white bread
- 1 tablespoon flat-leafed parsley (minced)
- 1 garlic clove (crushed)

- 1 1/2 tablespoons olive oil
- Ground black pepper

Directions/Instructions:

1. Put the bread slices in a food processor and process into fine crumbs. Add pepper, parsley, and garlic. Process until combined. Transfer to a bowl. Add olive oil and mix well.

2. Chop of the mushroom stalks. Scoop the crumb mixture into the mushroom caps and pat using your hands to make them stick.

3. Arrange the mushroom caps in the cooking basket. Cook for 8 minutes at 390 degrees.

Side Dishes

Cheese Sticks

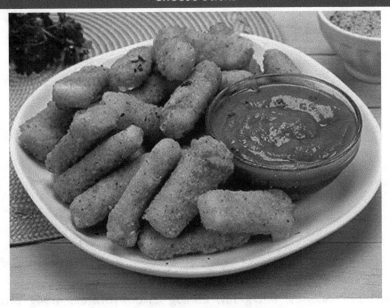

Nutritional Facts/Calories: 255 calories, 13.84g fat, 12.24g carbohydrates, 19.5g protein, 246mg cholesterol, 517mg sodium

Preparation + Cook Time: 30 minutes

Servings: 6

Ingredients:

- Marinara sauce for dipping
- 2 eggs (beaten)
- 1/4 cup grated Parmesan cheese
- 1/4 cup all-purpose flour
- 12 strings of part-skim mozzarella string cheese
- 2 cups breadcrumbs (Italian seasoned)

Directions/Instructions:

1. Separate the cheese strings and freeze for a couple of hours.

2. Mix to combine the Parmesan cheese and breadcrumbs in a shallow dish.

3. Beat the eggs in a bowl and transfer to a Ziploc bag. Add flour and the frozen cheese strings. Shake until coated.

4. Dip each string in the beaten egg and coat with the cheese and breadcrumbs mixture.

5. Arrange 6 pieces cheese string at a time in the cooking basket. Cook for 7 minutes at 400 degrees. Flip the cheese sticks and cook for 3 more minutes. Transfer to a platter and cook the rest of the cheese sticks.

6. Serve the cooked cheese sticks along with the dipping sauce.

Fried Avocado Tacos

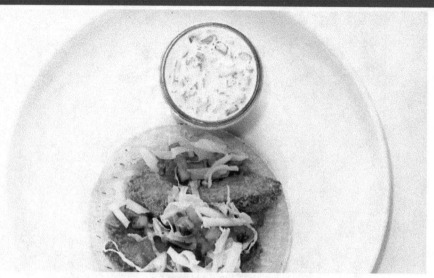

Nutritional Facts/Calories: 179 calories, 6.07g fat, 26.29g carbohydrates, 4.94g protein, 52mg cholesterol, 363mg sodium

Preparation + Cook Time: 20 minutes

Servings: 12

Ingredients:

- Tortillas and toppings
- 1 egg
- 1 avocado (divide and remove the seed)
- 1/2 cup panko breadcrumbs
- Salt to taste

Directions/Instructions:

1. Scoop out the meat from each avocado shell and slice them into wedges.

2. Beat the egg in a shallow bowl and put the breadcrumbs in another bowl.

3. Dip the avocado wedges in the beaten egg and coat with the breadcrumbs. Sprinkle them with a bit of salt. Arrange them in the cooking basket in a single layer.

4. Cook for 15 minutes at 392 degrees. Shake the basket halfway through the cooking process.

5. Put the cooked avocado wedges in tortillas and add your preferred toppings.

Roasted Heirloom Tomato with Baked Feta

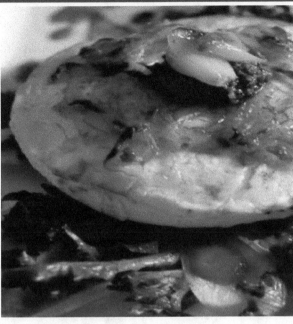

Nutritional Facts/Calories: 493 calories, 46.23g fat, 8.61g carbohydrates, 12.69g protein, 61mg cholesterol, 832mg sodium

Preparation + Cook Time: 34 minutes

Servings: 4

Ingredients:

- 1/2 cup red onions (thinly sliced)
- 1 8-ounce block of feta cheese
- 2 heirloom tomatoes

For the basil pesto

- 1/2 cup olive oil
- 1 garlic clove
- 3 tablespoons toasted pine nuts
- 1/2 cup basil (chopped)

- 1 tablespoon olive oil
- A pinch of salt

- 1/2 cup parsley (chopped)
- 1/2 cup grated parmesan cheese
- A pinch of salt

Directions/Instructions:

1. Prepare the pesto. Put the toasted pine nuts, garlic, salt, basil, and parmesan in a food processor. Process until combined. Gradually add oil as you mix. Process until everything is blended. Transfer to a bowl and cover. Refrigerate until ready to use.

2. Slice the feta and tomato into round slices with half an inch thickness. Use paper towels to pat them dry.

3. Spread a tablespoon of pesto on top of each tomato slice. Top with a slice of feta.

4. In a small bowl, mix a tablespoon of olive oil and the red onions. Scoop the mixture on top of the feta layer. Arrange them in the cooking basket. Cook for 14 minutes at 390 degrees.

5. Transfer to a platter and add a tablespoon of basil pesto on top of each. Sprinkle them with a bit of salt before serving.

Sweet Potato Fries

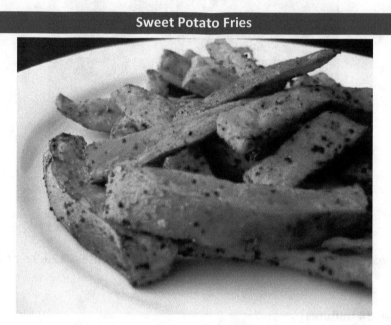

Nutritional Facts/Calories: 176 calories, 3.46g fat, 32.78g carbohydrates, 4.08g protein, 3mg cholesterol, 722mg sodium

Preparation + Cook Time: 45 minutes

Servings: 2

Ingredients:

- 1 sweet potato (rinsed and peeled)
- 1 tablespoon extra-virgin olive oil
- 1/2 teaspoon Cajun seasoning
- 1/2 teaspoon kosher salt
- 1 teaspoon Parmesan cheese (grated)

Directions/Instructions:

1. Slice the sweet potato into 1/4-inch thick sticks. Put them in a bowl. Add the remaining ingredients and toss until coated.

2. Arrange half of the fries in the cooking basket. Cook for 10 minutes at 400 degrees. Toss the fries halfway through the cooking process. Transfer the cooked fries to a platter and cook the remaining fries.

2. Season with salt and serve with your preferred dipping sauce.

Appetizer

Crispy Potato Skin Wedges

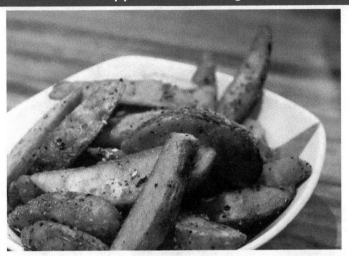

Nutritional Facts/Calories: 335 calories, 5.05g fat, 67.15g carbohydrates, 8.01g protein, 213mg sodium

Preparation + Cook Time: 56 minutes

Servings: 6

Ingredients:

- 2 tablespoons canola oil
- 1 1/2 teaspoons paprika
- 6 russet potatoes
- 1/2 teaspoon salt
- 1/2 teaspoon black pepper

Directions/Instructions:

1. Rinse the potatoes and scrub until clean. Put them in a pot with salted water. Boil for 40 minutes until tender. Leave to cool and refrigerate for 30 minutes.

2. In a bowl, mix salt, black pepper, paprika, and canola oil.

3. Slice the potatoes into quarters and put them in a bowl. Add the mixture of oil and spices. Toss until combined.

4. Arrange the potato wedges with the skin side facing down in the cooking basket. Cook for 16 minutes at 390 degrees.

Crunchy Eggplant Fries

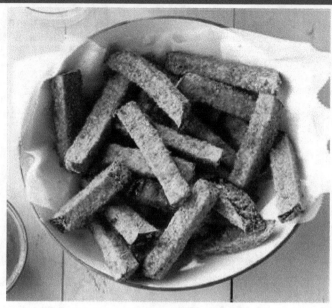

Nutritional Facts/Calories: 336 calories, 14.95g fat, 35.12g carbohydrates, 17.33g protein, 338mg cholesterol, 329mg sodium

Preparation + Cook Time: 20 minutes

Servings: 2

Ingredients:

- 2 tablespoons of milk
- Marinara for dipping
- 1 eggplant (peeled, cut lengthwise into slices and into 1/4-inch strips)
- 2 cups seasoned panko breadcrumbs
- 1 egg (beaten)
- 1/2 cup Italian cheese blend (shredded)

Directions/Instructions:

1. Whisk the egg and milk in a baking dish until combined.

2. Put cheese and panko breadcrumbs in another baking dish. Mix well.

3. Dip the eggplant slices in the egg mixture and coat them with the breadcrumb mixture.

4. Arrange an even layer of the coated eggplant slices in the cooking basket. Lightly spray them with oil. Cook for 5 minutes at 400 degrees. Transfer to a platter and cook the remaining eggplant slices.

5. Serve while warm along with the marinara sauce for dipping.

Easy Baked Mac and Cheese

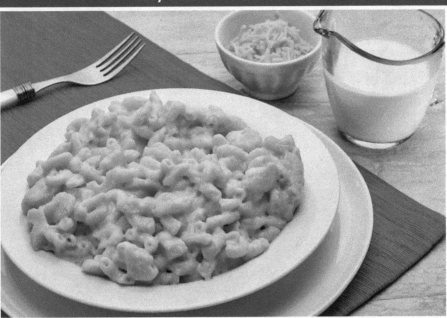

Nutritional Facts/Calories: 470 calories, 16.71g fat, 44.37g carbohydrates, 34.13g protein, 75mg cholesterol, 761mg sodium

Preparation + Cook Time: 19 minutes

Servings: 3

Ingredients:

- 1/2 cup mozzarella cheese (shredded)
- 1/4 cup Parmesan cheese (shredded)
- 3/4 cup cheddar cheese (shredded)
- 1 cup chicken broth
- 1 1/2 cups elbow macaroni
- Salt and pepper to taste
- 1/2 cup heavy cream

Directions/Instructions:

1. Put the macaroni in a pot with salted water. Lightly boil until half-cooked. This will take about 5 minutes. Drain the liquid and transfer to a bowl.

2. Add the remaining ingredients in the bowl with the cooked macaroni. Season with salt and pepper. Mix until combined. Transfer to a greased baking dish. Place the baking dish in the cooking basket. Cook for 30 minutes at 350 degrees.

Fried Mac and Cheese Balls

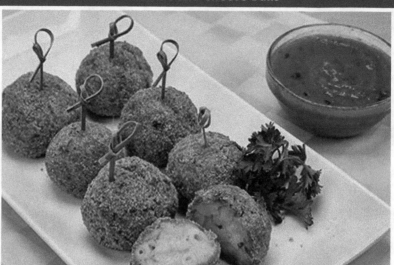

Nutritional Facts/Calories: 907 calories, 40.23g fat, 85.74g carbohydrates, 49.99g protein, 332mg cholesterol, 1980mg sodium

Preparation + Cook Time: 45 minutes

Servings: 6

Ingredients:

- 2 cups cream (heated), plus 2 tablespoons for the egg wash
- Salt and pepper to taste
- 2 tablespoons all-purpose flour
- 2 tablespoons unsalted butter
- 2 eggs

- 1 pound cheddar cheese (grated)
- 1 pound elbow macaroni
- 3 cups seasoned panko breadcrumbs
- 1/2 pound Parmesan cheese (shredded)
- 1/2 pound mozzarella cheese (shredded)

Directions/Instructions:

1. Cook the macaroni according to the package directions. Rinse with cold water and drain. Transfer to a bowl and set aside.

2. Melt butter in a saucepan over medium flame. Add flour and whisk for a couple of minutes. Stir the heated cream until there are no more lumps. Cook until thick. Remove from the stove. Stir in the cheeses until melted. Season with salt and pepper.

3. Pour the cheese mixture over the cooked macaroni. Gently fold until combined. Transfer to a shallow pan and refrigerate for 2 hours.

4. Use your hands to form meatball-sized balls from the mixture. Arrange them in a tray lined with wax paper. Freeze overnight.

5. Prepare the egg wash by combining 2 tablespoons of cream and eggs in a shallow bowl.

6. Dip the frozen mac and cheese balls in the egg wash and coat them with panko breadcrumbs. Gently press to make the coating stick. Arrange them in the cooking basket. Cook for 8 minutes at 400 degrees.

Grilled Cheese

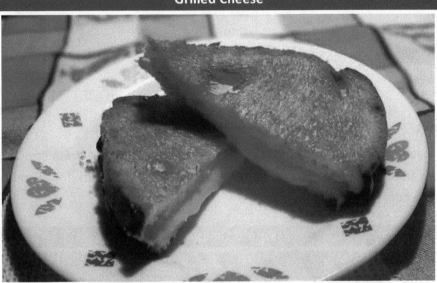

Nutritional Facts/Calories: 365 calories, 33g fat, 9.5g carbohydrates, 8.7g protein, 91mg cholesterol, 461mg sodium

Preparation + Cook Time: 27 minutes

Servings: 2

Ingredients:

- 1/4 cup melted butter
- 1/2 cup sharp cheddar cheese
- 4 slices of white bread or brioche

Directions/Instructions:

1. Put the cheese in a bowl and the butter in another bowl. Brush all sides of the bread slices with butter. Put cheese on top of 2 bread slices and cover each with the rest of the bread slices.

2. Arrange them in the cooking basket. Cook for 7 minutes at 360 degrees.

Kale Chips

Nutritional Facts/Calories: 127 calories, 13.65g fat, 1.4g carbohydrates, 0.68g protein, 1169mg sodium

Preparation + Cook Time: 15 minutes

Servings: 2

Ingredients:

- A bundle of kale
- 2 tablespoons olive oil
- 1 teaspoon sea salt

Directions/Instructions:

1. Chop off the kale leaves from the stems and trim. Rinse the leaves and pat them dry. Transfer to a bowl. Add salt and olive oil. Toss until combined. Put them in the cooking basket. Cook for 10 minutes at 400 degrees. Shake it once during the cooking process.

Potato Croquettes

Nutritional Facts/Calories: 704 calories, 25.26g fat, 96.52g carbohydrates, 24.57g protein, 423mg cholesterol, 597mg sodium

Preparation + Cook Time: 38 minutes

Servings: 4

Ingredients:

For the breading

- 2 eggs (beaten)
- 3/4 cup breadcrumbs
- 3/4 cup all-purpose flour
- 3 tablespoons vegetable oil

For the filling

- 2 egg yolks
- 4 russet potatoes (peeled and cut into cubes)
- Salt and pepper to taste
- Nutmeg to taste
- 1 cup grated Parmesan cheese
- 3 tablespoons chopped chives
- 2 tablespoons all-purpose flour

Directions/Instructions:

1. Put the cubed potatoes in a pot with salted water. Boil for 15 minutes. Drain the liquid. Transfer the potatoes to a bowl and mash. Leave to cool.

2. In another bowl, combine chives, cheese, flour, and egg yolks. Season with nutmeg, salt, and pepper. Add the mashed potato and mix until combined. Use your hands to form golf-size potato balls. Set them aside.

3. In a shallow bowl, combine the breadcrumbs and oil until loose.

4. Coat each potato ball with flour, dip in the beaten eggs and the oil and breadcrumbs mixture. Shape each coated ball into a cylinder.

5. Arrange the coated potato croquettes in the cooking basket. Cook for 8 minutes at 390 degrees.

Snacks

Barbeque Corn Sandwich

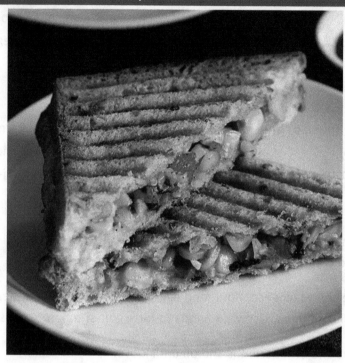

Nutritional Facts/Calories: 142 calories, 7.8g fat, 17.9g carbohydrates, 2.4g protein, 15mg cholesterol, 357mg sodium

Preparation + Cook Time: 45 minutes

Servings: 4

Ingredients:

- 1 capsicum
- 1 cup sweet corn kernels
- 2 tablespoon butter (room temperature)

For the sauce

- 1/3 cup stock or water
- 1/4 teaspoon mustard powder
- Salt and black pepper to taste
- 1 1/2 tablespoons tomato ketchup
- 1/4 cup onion (chopped)

- 4 slices of white bread (cut the edges and slice the bread horizontally)

- 1 teaspoon olive oil
- 1 garlic flake (crushed)
- 1/2 tablespoon sugar
- 1/2 tablespoon Worcestershire sauce
- 1/2 tablespoon red chili sauce

Directions/Instructions:

1. Heat oil in a pan over medium-high flame. Add garlic and onions and cook for 4 minutes while stirring often. Add the sugar, chili sauce, mustard, stock, Worcestershire sauce, and tomato ketchup. Mix well and bring to a boil. Turn the heat to low and simmer for 10 minutes. Season with salt and black pepper. Set aside.

2. Place another pan over medium flame. Melt butter and roast the corn kernels.

3. Lightly rub a bit of oil on the capsicum. Roast and turn them over until black patches develop. Remove the skin and seeds. Chop it finely and transfer to a bowl. Add the barbecue sauce and roasted corn kernels. Mix well. Spread the mixture on a slice of bread and put another slice on top.

4. Put the sandwich in the cooking basket. Cook for 15 minutes at 356 degrees. Flip the sandwich halfway through the cooking process.

5. Serve along with chutney while hot.

Corn Bread

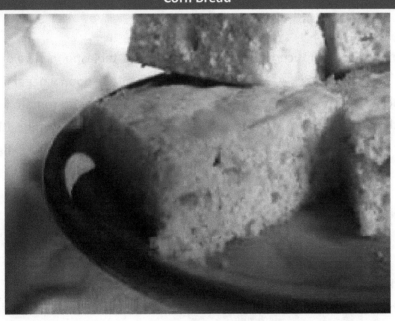

Nutritional Facts/Calories: 372 calories, 20.16g fat, 39.04g carbohydrates, 8.87g protein, 312mg cholesterol, 395mg sodium

Preparation + Cook Time: 30 minutes

Servings: 4

Ingredients:

- 1/2 cup whole milk
- 1/2 cup all-purpose flour
- 1/2 teaspoon kosher salt
- 1/4 cup vegetable oil
- 1/2 cup corn kernels (fresh or frozen)
- 1/2 cup yellow cornmeal
- 2 tablespoons sugar
- 2 eggs
- 1 1/2 teaspoons baking powder

Directions/Instructions:

1. Combine all the dry ingredients in a bowl and whisk.

2. In another bowl, put all the wet ingredient. Gently mix until combined. Gradually add the dry mixture into the bowl. Mix until smooth. Add the corn and mix until combined.

3. Transfer the mixture into a greased baking dish. Put it in the cooking basket. Cook for 25 minutes at 350 degrees.

4. Allow to cool before transferring to a plate. Slice and serve.

Corn Rolls

Nutritional Facts/Calories: 510 calories, 30g fat, 32.5g carbohydrates, 16g protein

Preparation + Cook Time: 50 minutes

Servings: 4

Ingredients:

- 3 tablespoons of 3 colored capsicums (finely chopped)
- 1 cup cream-style corn
- 1 onion (finely chopped)
- Salt and pepper to taste
- 1 tablespoon olive oil
- 1 teaspoon vinegar
- 1 teaspoon tomato ketchup
- 1 green chili (minced)
- 4 bread slices (cut the sides)

For sealing paste

- 2 teaspoons maida (dissolved in 2 teaspoons of water)

For garnishing

- 1 teaspoon black sesame seeds
- 1 tablespoon white sesame seeds

Directions/Instructions:

1. Heat oil in a pan over medium-high flame. Put the onions and cook for 3 minutes. Stir in the capsicums, green chili, ketchup, pepper, salt, vinegar, and corn. Cook for 4 minutes while stirring often. Transfer to a bowl and leave to cool.

2. Flatten the bread slices using a rolling pin. Place the corn mixture near the edge of each bread slice. Roll it tightly until the filling is covered. Seal the ends with the prepared sealing paste. Lightly wet the rolls with water. Coat them with sesame seeds. Repeat the step with the rest of the bread slices and filling. Arrange in a tray. Wrap with a cling film and refrigerate.

4. Divide each roll into 2. Put them in the cooking basket. Cook for 20 minutes at 320 degrees. Flip the rolls halfway through the cooking process.

5. Serve while hot. Garnish with lemon wedges and use hot sauce for dipping.

French Fries

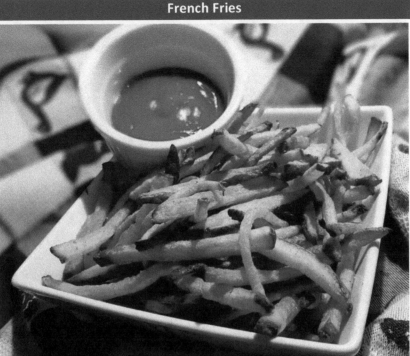

Nutritional Facts/Calories: 497 calories, 7.19g fat, 100g carbohydrates, 11.84g protein, 28mg sodium

Preparation + Cook Time: 1 hour 10 minutes

Servings: 4

Ingredients:

- 6 russet potatoes (peeled)
- 2 tablespoons olive oil

Directions/Instructions:

1. Slice the peeled potatoes into strips. Soak them in water for half an hour. Drain and pat excess moisture with paper towels. Put them in a bowl and add oil. Toss until coated.

2. Put the potato slices in the cooking basket. Cook for 30 minutes at 360 degrees. Shake twice during the cooking process.

Grilled Scallion Cheese Sandwich

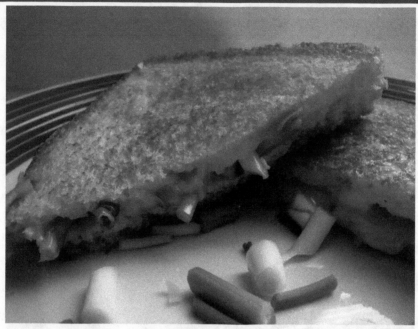

Nutritional Facts/Calories: 511 calories, 39.4g fat, 12.9g carbohydrates, 27.6g protein, 119mg cholesterol, 838mg sodium

Preparation + Cook Time: 20 minutes

Servings: 1

Ingredients:

- 2 teaspoons butter (room temperature)
- 3/4 cup grated cheddar cheese
- 2 slices of bread
- 1 tablespoon grated parmesan cheese
- 2 scallions (thinly sliced)

Directions/Instructions:

1. Spread a teaspoon of butter on a slice of bread. Place it in the cooking basket with the buttered side facing down. Add scallions and cheddar cheese on top. Spread the rest of the butter in the other slice of bread. Place it on top of the sandwich and sprinkle with Parmesan cheese.

2. Cook for 10 minutes at 356 degrees.

Snack Mix

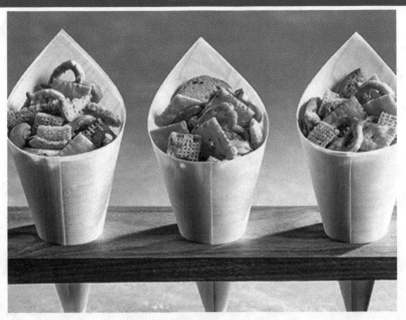

Nutritional Facts/Calories: 518 calories, 27g fat, 50.97g carbohydrates, 22.7g protein, 30mg cholesterol, 475mg sodium

Preparation + Cook Time: 25 minutes

Servings: 6

Ingredients:

- 2 tablespoons melted butter
- 1 tablespoon Worcestershire sauce
- 6 cups mixed cereal
- 1 cup peanuts
- 1 cup small cheese crackers
- A pinch of salt

Directions/Instructions:

1. Put the Worcestershire sauce, melted butter, and salt in a bowl. Mix well. Add the nuts, crackers, and cereals, and stir. Transfer the mixture to the cooking basket. Cook for 15 minutes at 320 degrees. Stir the mix every 5 minutes.

2. Transfer to a bowl and leave to cool. Store in an airtight container.

Desserts

Apricot Blackberry Crumble

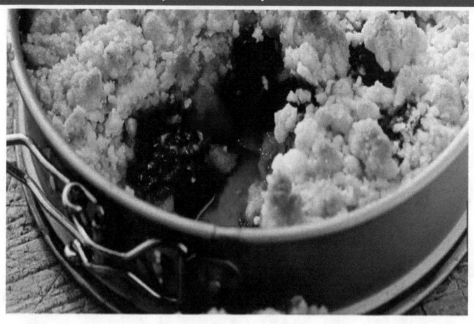

Nutritional Facts/Calories: 217 calories, 7.44g fat, 36.2g carbohydrates, 2.3g protein, 19mg cholesterol, 80mg sodium

Preparation + Cook Time: 30 minutes

Servings: 8

Ingredients:

- 5.5 ounces fresh blackberries
- 18 ounces fresh apricots (remove the seeds and cut into cubes)
- Salt to taste

- 2 tablespoons lemon juice
- 5 tablespoons cold butter
- 1 cup flour
- 1/2 cup sugar

Directions/Instructions:

1. Put the apricots and blackberries in a bowl. Add lemon juice and 2 tablespoons of sugar. Mix until combined. Transfer the mixture to a baking dish.

2. Put flour, the rest of the sugar, and a pinch of salt in a bowl. Mix well. Add a tablespoon of cold butter. Use your hands to combine the mixture until it becomes crumbly. Put this on top of the fruit mixture and press it down lightly.

3. Place the baking dish in the cooking basket. Cook for 20 minutes at 390 degrees.

4. Allow to cool before slicing and serving.

Chocolate Cake Version 1

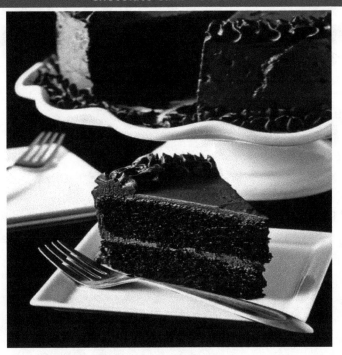

Nutritional Facts/Calories: 377 calories, 14.62g fat, 57g carbohydrates, 5.58g protein, 294mg sodium

Preparation + Cook Time: 35 minutes

Servings: 4

Ingredients:

- 1 cup water
- 3/4 cup granulated sugar
- 1 tablespoon white vinegar
- 1 teaspoon baking soda
- 1 teaspoon pure vanilla extract

- 1/4 cup vegetable oil
- 1/2 teaspoon kosher salt
- 3 tablespoons cocoa powder (unsweetened)
- 1 1/2 cups all-purpose flour

Directions/Instructions:

1. Put all the ingredients in a bowl. Mix using a hand mixer at a low-speed setting until combined. Transfer the batter to a greased baking dish.

2. Put the baking dish in the cooking basket. Cook for 30 minutes at 330 degrees.

3. Top with whipped cream and serve while warm.

Chocolate Cake Version 2

Nutritional Facts/Calories: 333 calories, 14.48g fat, 46.2g carbohydrates, 5.58g protein, 208mg cholesterol, 59mg sodium

Preparation + Cook Time: 50 minutes

Servings: 10

Ingredients:

- 6 tablespoons cocoa powder
- 1/2 teaspoon baking soda
- 1 teaspoon baking powder
- 9 tablespoons unsalted butter
- 2/3 cup caster sugar

- 2 teaspoons vanilla
- 1/2 cup sour cream
- 1 cup flour
- 3 eggs

For the chocolate icing:

- 5.5 ounces chocolate
- 1 teaspoon vanilla
- 1 2/3 cups icing sugar

- 3 1/2 tablespoons unsalted butter (room temperature)

Directions/Instructions:

1. Put all the ingredients for the cake in a food processor. Process until combined. Transfer to a baking dish.

2. Put the baking dish in the cooking basket. Cook for 35 minutes at 320 degrees. Transfer to a wire rack and leave to cool.

3. Melt the chocolate in the microwave. Let it cool down a bit before adding to the remaining ingredients for the icing.

4. Transfer the cake to a plate. Spread the icing all over. Slice and serve.

Chocolate Marshmallow Bread Pudding

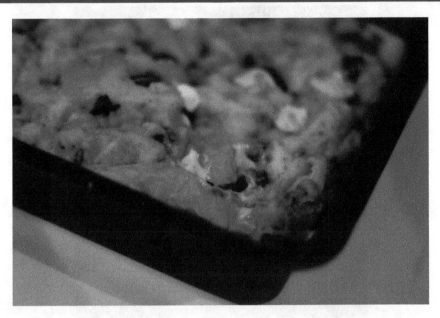

Nutritional Facts/Calories: 741 calories, 48.5g fat, 60.23g carbohydrates, 15.6g protein, 751mg cholesterol, 626mg sodium

Preparation + Cook Time: 55 minutes

Servings: 4

Ingredients:

- 2 1/2 cups heavy cream
- 1 teaspoon pure vanilla extract
- 1 teaspoon fresh lemon juice
- 1/2 cup mini marshmallows
- 3/4 cup sugar

- 1/4 cup chocolate chips
- 1/2 teaspoon kosher salt
- 4 eggs
- 5 croissants (sliced into 1-inch cubes)

Directions/Instructions:

1. Put the eggs, cream, lemon juice, salt, vanilla extract, and sugar in a blender. Process until smooth.

2. Arrange the cubed croissant in the cooking basket. Cook for 5 minutes at 400 degrees.

3. Soak the toasted croissant cubes in the custard mixture. Transfer the mixture to a greased baking dish. Add the marshmallows and chocolate chips. Gently stir.

4. Put the baking dish in the cooking basket. Cook for 25 minutes at 340 degrees.

5. Top with whipped cream and serve while warm.

Vanilla Soufflé

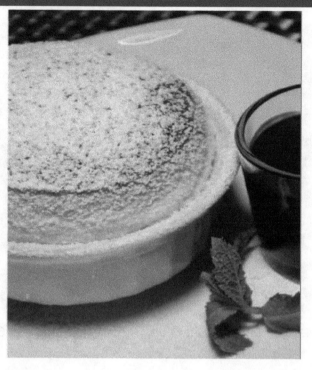

Nutritional Facts/Calories: 215 calories, 12.2g fat, 18.98g carbohydrates, 6.66g protein, 148mg cholesterol, 131mg sodium

Preparation + Cook Time: 52 minutes

Servings: 6

Ingredients:

- 1/4 cup softened butter
- 1/4 cup sugar
- 1/4 cup all-purpose flour
- 5 egg whites
- 4 egg yolks

- 1 teaspoon cream of tartar
- 2 teaspoons vanilla extract
- 1 vanilla bean
- 1-ounce sugar
- 1 cup whole milk

Directions/Instructions:

1. Mix the butter and flour in a bowl until the mixture becomes a smooth paste.

2. Heat milk in a pan over medium flame. Add sugar and stir until dissolved. Add the vanilla bean and bring to a boil. Beat the mixture using a wire whisk as you add the butter and flour mixture. Continue whisking until there are no more lumps. Reduce the heat to low and simmer until thick. Discard the vanilla bean. Turn off the heat.

3. Place them on an ice bath and allow to cool for 10 minutes.

4. Grease 6 ramekins with butter. Sprinkle each with a bit of sugar.

5. Beat the egg yolks in a bowl. Add the vanilla extract and milk mixture. Mix until combined.

6. In another bowl, beat the egg whites, cream of tartar and sugar until it forms medium stiff peaks. Gradually fold the egg whites into the soufflé base. Transfer the mixture to the ramekins.

7. Put 3 ramekins in the cooking basket at a time. Cook for 16 minutes at 330 degrees. Transfer to a wire rack to cool and cook the rest.

8. Sprinkle powdered sugar on top and drizzle with chocolate sauce before serving.

Conclusion

I hope this book was able to help you to understand the benefits of an Air Fryer and the basics on how to use it. The next step is to plan your meals and gather the ingredients. This appliance is easy to use and you will eventually get the hang of the process. Once you have tried several recipes, you can already start tweaking the ingredients to create variations or start making your own. Enjoy the process of preparing your meals in a healthier way using this innovation when it comes to cooking.

For even more delicious and colorful recipes not covered in this book, check out other books in the Air Fryer Recipe Series by Barbara Trisler!

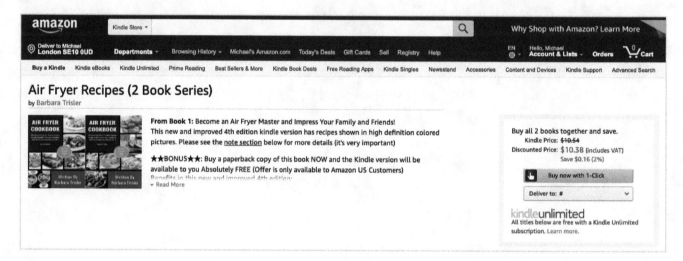

The End

Thank you very much for taking the time to read this book. I tried my best to cover as many air fryer recipes as possible. If you found it useful please let me know by leaving a review on Amazon! Your support really does make a difference and I read all the reviews personally so can I understand what my readers particularly enjoyed and then feature more of that in future books.

I also pride myself on giving my readers the best information out there, being super responsive to them and providing the best customer service. If you feel I have fallen short of this standard in any way, please kindly email me at BarbaraTrisler@yahoo.com so I can get a chance to make it right to you.

I wish you all the best!

Glossary

Note – If the recipe you're interested in is not in this book 1, it might be in book 2 of this "Air Fryer Recipe" series

CPSIA information can be obtained
at www.ICGtesting.com
Printed in the USA
LVHW062007130723
752301LV00007B/209